THE PALEO DIET FOOD GUIDE

The ultimate guide to eating the primary way

By

Candice Foster

Table of contents

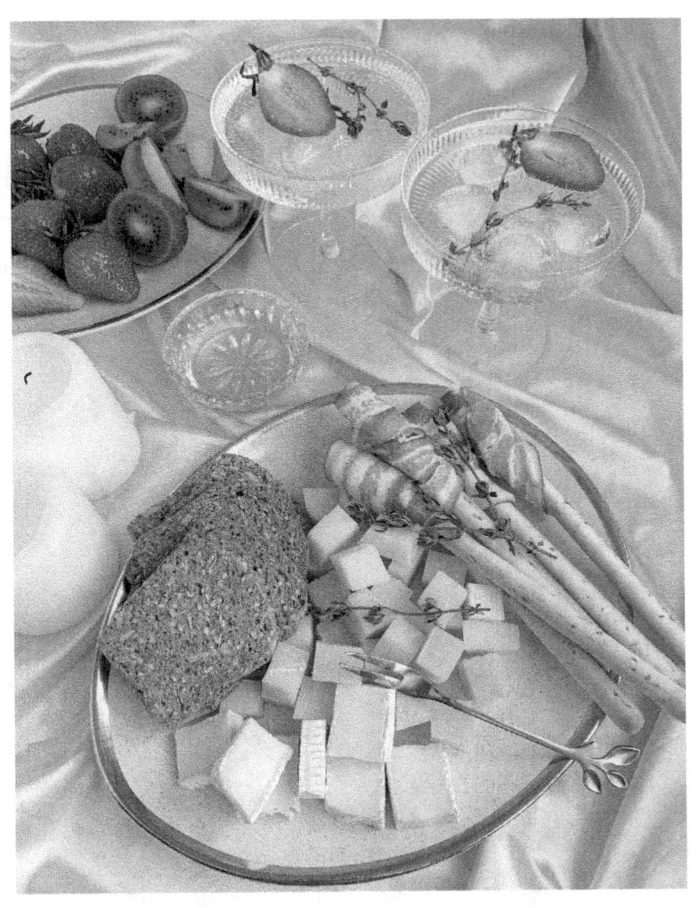

INTRODUCTION

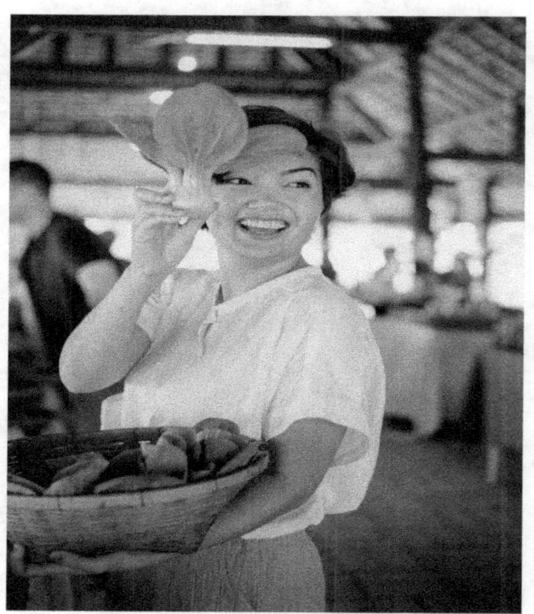

The Paleo food guide, a modern adaptation of the presumed dietary habits of early humans, has gained substantial popularity in recent years. This dietary regimen revolves around the premise that our bodies are inherently better suited to the foods our Paleolithic ancestors consumed over 10,000 years ago, before the advent of agriculture. Central to the Paleo food guide are unprocessed, nutrient-dense foods, mirroring those that could have been gathered or hunted in the wild, such as lean meats, fish, fruits, vegetables, nuts, and seeds. The elimination of processed foods, grains, legumes, and dairy is a defining characteristic of this regimen. Proponents of the Paleo diet advocate that by adhering to this ancestral eating pattern, individuals may experience various health benefits, including improved weight management, enhanced blood sugar regulation, and better overall metabolic health. Moreover, the emphasis on whole foods with minimal additives aligns with contemporary nutritional recommendations for promoting general wellness and preventing chronic diseases. Despite its growing popularity, the Paleo diet has faced scrutiny from some health professionals, who highlight potential nutritional deficiencies and the exclusion of certain food groups, raising concerns about the sustainability and long-term feasibility of this dietary approach. This introduction aims to examine the underlying principles, potential advantages, and criticisms associated with the Paleo food guide, offering a comprehensive overview of this contentious yet intriguing dietary philosophy.

Historical Background of the Paleo diet.

The paleo diet, also known as the Paleolithic diet or caveman diet, is based on the idea of eating foods similar to those consumed by our ancient ancestors during the Paleolithic era. This diet emphasizes consuming whole foods, such as lean meats, fish, fruits, vegetables, nuts, and seeds, while avoiding processed foods, grains, dairy, and refined sugars. It gained popularity in the 21st century, with its origins rooted in the evolutionary premise that our bodies are best adapted to the diet of early humans. Proponents of the paleo diet argue that it promotes weight loss, improved blood sugar control, and other health benefits by mimicking the dietary patterns of our prehistoric ancestors. However, its effectiveness and long-term health impacts are still subjects of debate among nutritionists and health experts.

Principles and Philosophy of the Paleo diet.

The Paleo diet, also known as the Paleolithic diet is centered around the idea of consuming foods similar to those eaten by our ancient ancestors. It operates on the principle that the human body is genetically mismatched to modern diets, which often include processed foods, grains, and dairy. Instead, the Paleo diet focuses on whole, unprocessed foods that would have been available to early humans such as lean meats, fish, fruits, vegetables, nuts, and seeds.

Philosophically, the Paleo diet emphasizes a return to a more natural and primal way of eating, aiming to optimize health and prevent modern diet-related diseases. By eschewing processed foods and grains, proponents believe that individuals can reduce inflammation, improve digestion, and promote overall well-being. This philosophy is rooted in the belief that our bodies are best adapted to the foods that our ancestors evolved to eat over millions of years.

The Paleo diet is often criticized for its restrictive nature and for potentially excluding certain nutritious food groups. Critics argue that modern humans have evolved to tolerate a wider variety of foods and that the diet might not be suitable for everyone. Nonetheless, many proponents of the Paleo diet continue to advocate for its potential benefits in improving overall health and well-being.

CHAPTER 1

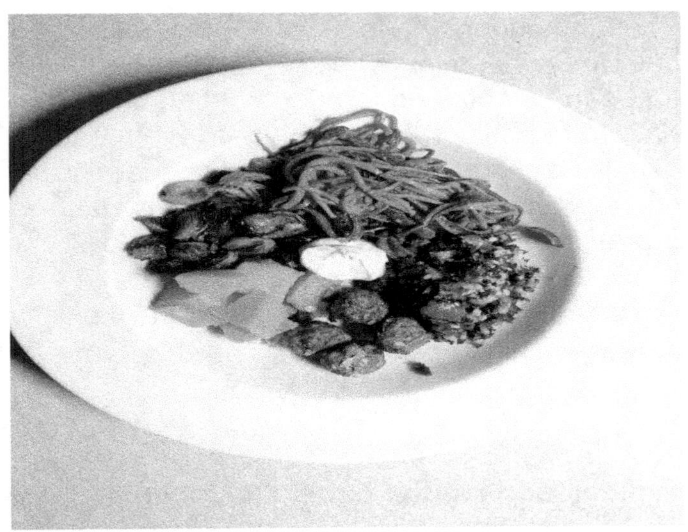

The Basics of the Paleo Diet; what to eat and what to avoid.

The paleo diet, also referred to as the Paleolithic diet, Stone Age diet, or caveman diet, is a dietary plan inspired by the presumed eating habits of early humans who lived during the Paleolithic era, a period that ended about

10,000 years ago. Proponents of the paleo diet believe that our bodies are genetically adapted to the diet of our ancient ancestors and that modern dietary changes, such as the introduction of processed foods, grains, and dairy, have contributed to the rise of chronic diseases.

The fundamental principle of the paleo diet involves consuming whole, unprocessed foods that can be obtained through hunting and gathering. This primarily includes lean meats, fish, fruits, vegetables, nuts, and seeds. The diet typically excludes grains, legumes, dairy products, refined sugar, and processed oils. While there is no one-size-fits-all approach to the paleo diet, the emphasis is generally on nutrient-dense, high-quality foods.

Typical foods in the paleo diet include:

Lean meats: These comprise game, poultry, and beef raised on grass.

Fish and seafood: Wild-caught fish and shellfish are recommended for their omega-3 fatty acids.
Fruits: Fresh fruits, in moderation, provide essential vitamins, minerals, and fiber.

Vegetables: Non-starchy vegetables, such as leafy greens, root vegetables, and cruciferous vegetables, are a staple of the paleo diet.
Nuts and seeds: These are a source of healthy fats, protein, and various essential nutrients.

Foods to avoid on the paleo diet include:

Grains: This includes wheat, oats, barley, and rice.
Legumes: Beans, lentils, and peanuts are typically excluded due to their lectin and phytate content.
Dairy: Milk, cheese, and yogurt are generally not part of the paleo diet, although some versions allow for grass-fed butter and ghee.
Refined sugar: Sugary beverages, pastries, and other processed foods containing added sugars are avoided.
Processed oils: Industrial seed oils like soybean oil, corn oil, and canola oil are replaced with healthier alternatives such as olive oil, coconut oil, and avocado oil. Advocates of the paleo diet claim various health benefits, including weight loss, improved blood sugar control, better appetite management, and reduced inflammation. However, some critics argue that the restrictive nature of the diet may lead to nutrient deficiencies, particularly in calcium and vitamin D, and that the scientific evidence supporting

its long-term efficacy and health benefits is
limited.

As with any diet, consulting a healthcare
provider or a registered dietitian before making
significant dietary changes is recommended to
ensure that the paleo diet is suitable for
individual health needs and goals. Additionally,
it's important to focus on a balanced approach
that emphasizes a variety of nutrient-rich foods
to support overall health and well-being.

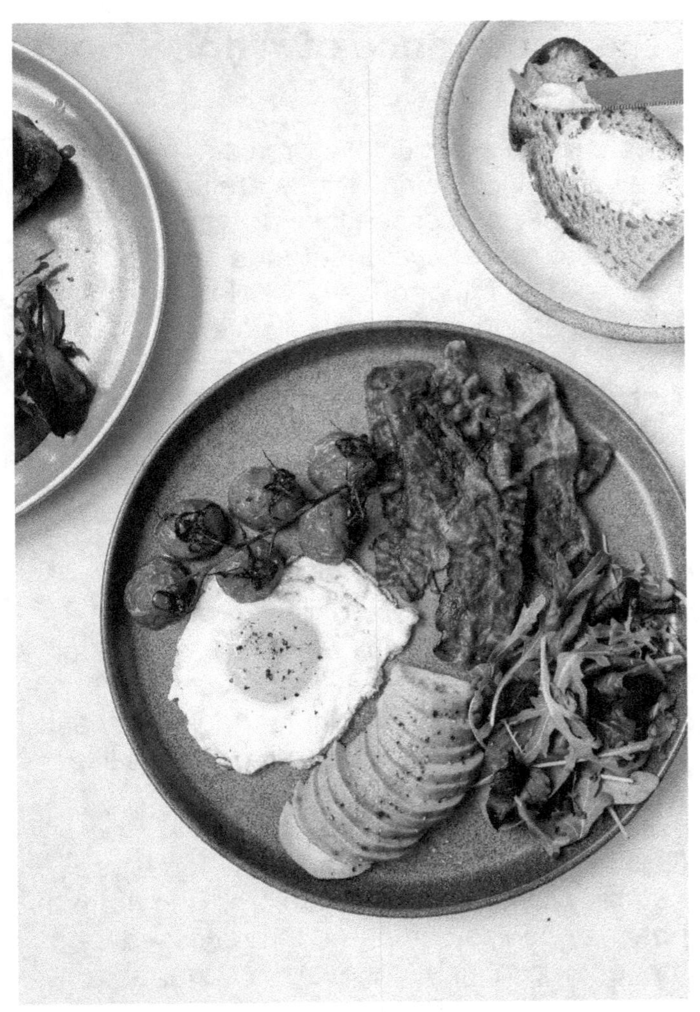

The Importance of Whole Foods

Whole foods are crucial for maintaining good health and well-being. These are unprocessed or minimally processed foods that are in their natural state or have undergone minimal refining. The importance of whole foods can be summarized in several key points:

Nutrient Density: Whole foods are rich in essential nutrients such as vitamins, minerals, fiber, and antioxidants. They provide a wide range of nutrients that are vital for the body's proper functioning.

Fiber Content: Whole foods are excellent sources of dietary fiber, which is essential for digestive health. Fiber helps prevent constipation, aids in weight management, and may reduce the risk of chronic diseases like heart disease and type 2 diabetes.

Reduced Added Sugars: Whole foods are naturally low in added sugars, making them a healthier choice compared to processed foods that often contain high levels of sugar and unhealthy sweeteners.

Satiety: Whole foods are more filling and satisfying than processed alternatives, which can help with weight management by reducing overeating and snacking.

Better Blood Sugar Control: Whole foods typically have a lower glycemic index, which means they have a gentler impact on blood sugar levels.
Those who currently have diabetes or are at risk of getting it should pay particular attention to this.

Lower Processed Additives: Whole foods are free from many of the additives, preservatives, and artificial ingredients found in processed foods. Avoiding these additives can help reduce health risks associated with their consumption.

Improved Heart Health: A diet rich in whole foods, such as fruits, vegetables, whole grains, and lean proteins, is associated with a lower risk of heart disease due to its favorable effects on blood pressure and cholesterol levels.

Weight Management: Incorporating whole foods into your diet can make it easier to maintain a healthy weight since they are less calorie-dense and more filling than processed options.

Variety and Taste: Whole foods offer a wide range of flavors, textures, and tastes. This diversity can make your meals more enjoyable and encourage a balanced diet.

Sustainability: Choosing whole foods, especially locally grown and seasonal options, can be more environmentally sustainable since they typically require fewer resources and have a smaller carbon footprint compared to heavily processed foods.

In summary, whole foods provide a wealth of health benefits, including better nutrition, weight management, and reduced risk of chronic diseases. By prioritizing whole foods in your diet, you can enhance your overall health and well-being while supporting sustainable and mindful eating habits.

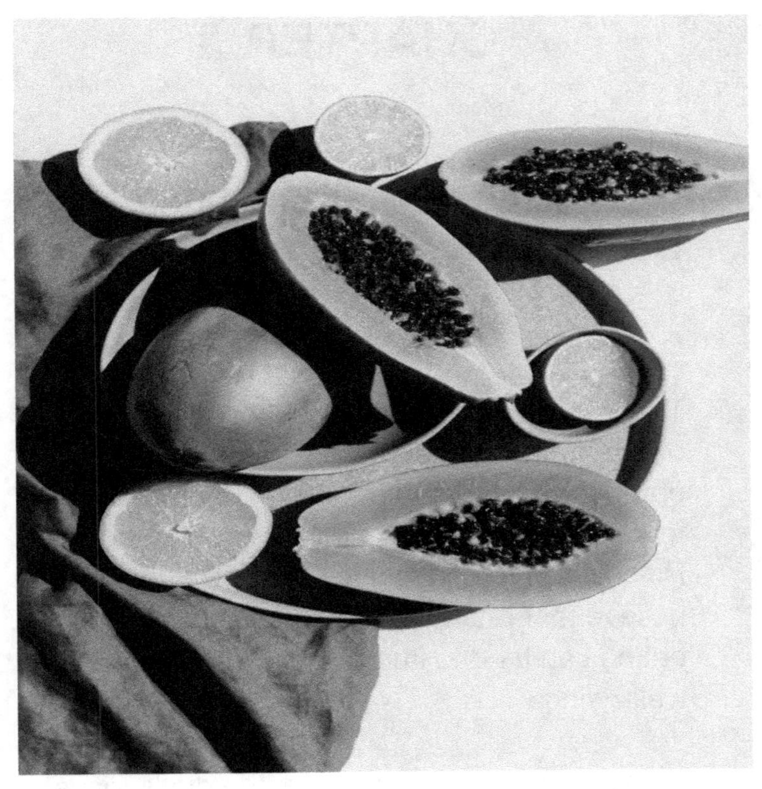

CHAPTER 2

Understanding the Science Behind Paleo diet.

The Paleo diet, is inspired by the dietary habits of our hunter-gatherer ancestors. It emphasizes consuming whole, unprocessed foods similar to those available during the Paleolithic era. Advocates of the Paleo diet believe that returning to this ancient way of eating can lead to improved health and well-being.

From a scientific perspective, the diet's focus on unprocessed foods, lean meats, fish, fruits, vegetables, nuts, and seeds aligns with recommendations for a healthy diet. It encourages the avoidance of processed foods, sugar, grains, and dairy, which may help reduce inflammation and stabilize blood sugar levels.

Research has shown that adhering to a Paleo diet can lead to weight loss, improved glucose tolerance, and better blood pressure control. However, some scientists express concerns about potential nutrient deficiencies, especially in terms of calcium and vitamin D due to the exclusion of dairy products.

While the Paleo diet has its benefits, individual variation, lifestyle, and specific health goals should be considered when adopting any dietary plan. Understanding the science behind the Paleo diet involves recognizing its potential benefits while being mindful of potential nutritional gaps and ensuring a balanced intake of essential nutrients.

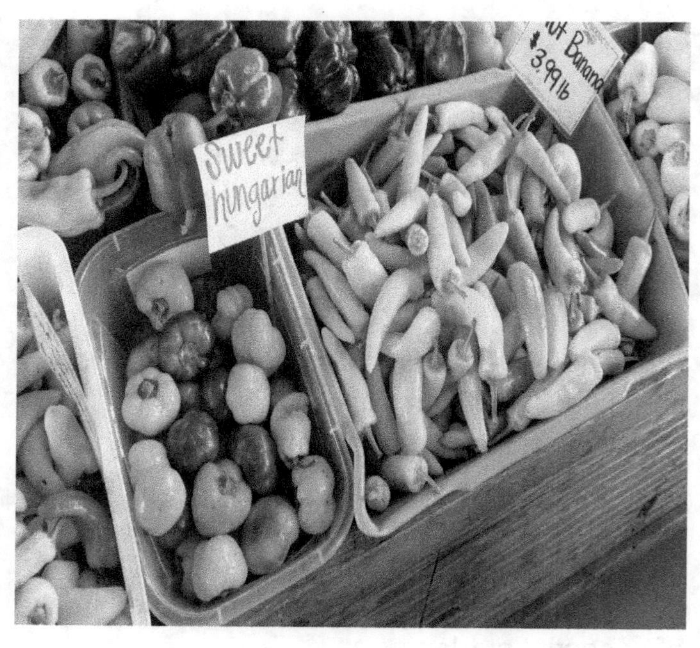
Sweet
hungarian
ut Banana
$3.99 lb

Evolutionary Biology and Nutrition

Evolutionary biology and nutrition form the core of the Paleo diet concept. Proponents of this dietary approach argue that our genetic makeup is best suited to the foods consumed by our Paleolithic ancestors. They emphasize that our bodies have not fully adapted to the dietary changes brought about by agriculture and modern food processing.

From an evolutionary biology perspective, the Paleo diet aligns with the idea that our ancestors primarily consumed lean meats, fish, fruits, vegetables, nuts, and seeds. This diet provided essential nutrients, healthy fats, and a balance of proteins and carbohydrates crucial for survival.

Nutritionally, the Paleo diet's emphasis on whole, unprocessed foods contributes to increased intake of fiber, vitamins, and minerals, while minimizing the consumption of refined sugars, processed foods, and grains. This dietary pattern may reduce the risk of chronic diseases, such as obesity, diabetes, and heart disease, which have become more prevalent in modern societies.

However, critics argue that the concept of replicating a historical diet overlooks the evolutionary changes that have occurred since the Paleolithic era. Human populations have adapted to diverse diets over time, which suggests that a single, ideal dietary pattern may not suit everyone. Furthermore, the exclusion of certain food groups, such as dairy and grains, may pose potential challenges in meeting specific nutritional needs.

Understanding the evolutionary biology and nutritional principles behind the Paleo diet involves recognizing the benefits of whole, unprocessed foods while acknowledging the need for a personalized, balanced approach to nutrition that accommodates individual variations and requirements.

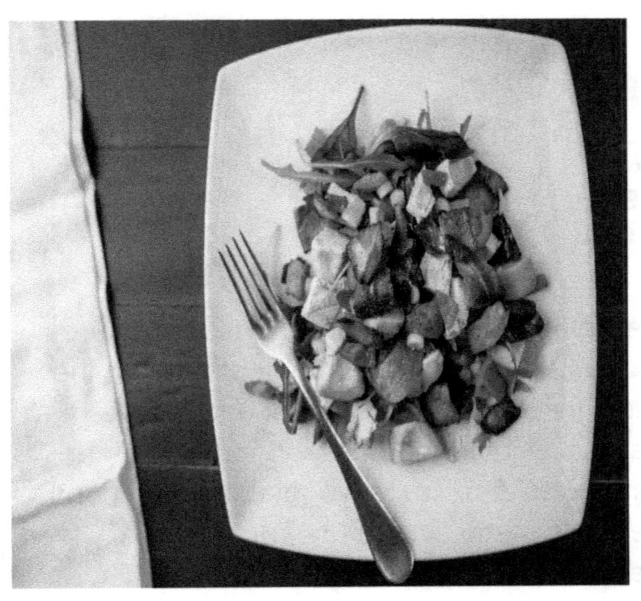

Health Implications of the Paleo diet.

The Paleo diet emphasizes consuming foods that our ancestors purportedly ate during the Paleolithic era. While this diet encourages the intake of whole, unprocessed foods such as lean meats, fish, fruits, vegetables, nuts, and seeds, its restrictive nature can potentially lead to certain health implications.

One possible concern is the exclusion of entire food groups, such as grains, dairy, and legumes, which may lead to nutrient deficiencies if not carefully monitored. Moreover, the high consumption of animal proteins in the Paleo diet might increase the risk of cardiovascular diseases and kidney problems over the long term. Additionally, the emphasis on red meats could potentially raise the risk of certain cancers.

Furthermore, due to the limitations imposed by the diet, individuals may find it challenging to meet their daily fiber requirements, which could lead to digestive issues such as constipation. It's important to consult a healthcare professional or a registered dietitian before adopting any restrictive diet to ensure it aligns with individual health goals and needs.

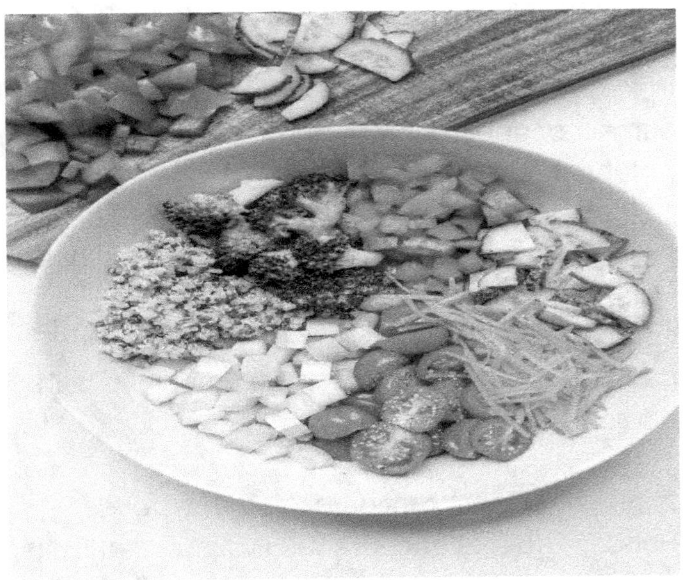

CHAPTER 3

Health Benefits of the Paleo diet

The Paleo diet, modeled after the presumed dietary patterns of our Paleolithic ancestors, emphasizes whole, unprocessed foods and excludes grains, legumes, and dairy. While its efficacy and long-term health impacts remain a subject of debate, proponents suggest several potential health benefits:

Weight Management: The emphasis on whole foods, lean protein, and healthy fats may contribute to weight loss and improved body composition, particularly when combined with an active lifestyle.

Increased Consumption of Nutrient-Dense Foods: The diet encourages the intake of fruits, vegetables, lean meats, fish, nuts, and seeds, which are rich in essential nutrients, vitamins, and minerals. This may promote general wellbeing and health.

Blood Sugar Regulation: By eliminating refined sugars and processed carbohydrates, the Paleo diet may help regulate blood sugar levels and improve insulin sensitivity, potentially benefiting individuals with diabetes or insulin resistance.

Reduced Inflammation: Some adherents report a reduction in inflammation-related conditions, such as arthritis and autoimmune diseases, due to the exclusion of processed foods and the focus on anti-inflammatory foods.

Improved Digestive Health: The diet's emphasis on high-fiber foods, including fruits, vegetables, and nuts, can promote a healthy digestive system, prevent constipation, and support a diverse gut microbiome.

Enhanced Heart Health: By avoiding processed foods and trans fats, and by focusing on sources of healthy fats (such as avocados and olive oil) and lean proteins, the Paleo diet may help lower the risk of heart disease and improve overall cardiovascular health.

Allergen Elimination: Excluding common allergenic foods like dairy and gluten may provide relief for individuals with sensitivities or intolerances, potentially reducing allergic reactions and digestive discomfort.

Increased Satiety: The diet's emphasis on protein, healthy fats, and fiber-rich foods can promote a feeling of fullness, potentially reducing overall calorie intake and aiding in appetite control.

Balanced Omega-3 to Omega-6 Ratio: Incorporating fatty fish, such as salmon, and various nuts and seeds can help achieve a healthier balance of omega-3 and omega-6 fatty acids, which is linked to improved cardiovascular and cognitive health.

While these potential benefits are often cited, it's important to note that the Paleo diet isn't without its criticisms. Critics argue that the exclusion of entire food groups may lead to nutritional deficiencies, and some aspects of the diet are still subject to ongoing scientific research and discussion. It's crucial to consult with a healthcare professional or registered dietitian before making significant dietary changes to ensure that individual nutritional needs are met.

Weight Management and Satiety

Weight management and satiety are critical components of a healthy lifestyle. When it comes to weight management, it's essential to strike a balance between the calories consumed and those expended. Incorporating a well-rounded diet rich in fruits, vegetables, whole grains, lean proteins, and healthy fats can help maintain a healthy weight. Additionally, staying physically active through regular exercise is crucial for achieving weight management goals.

Satiety, or the feeling of fullness, plays a key role in controlling food intake and preventing overeating. Including high-fiber foods, such as fruits, vegetables, and whole grains, can help promote satiety and prevent excessive calorie consumption. Additionally, consuming protein-rich foods can also contribute to a feeling of fullness and aid in weight management efforts. It's important to listen to your body's hunger and fullness cues and practice mindful eating to prevent unnecessary overconsumption.

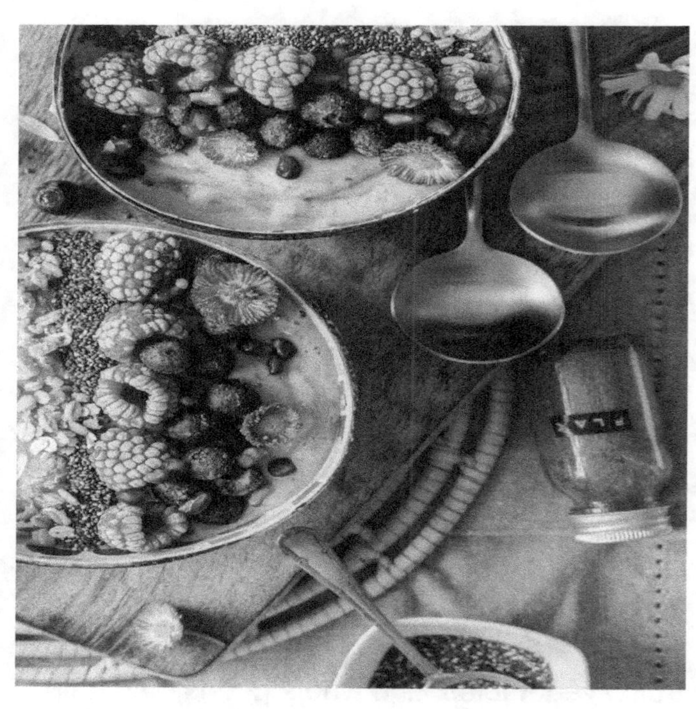

Improved Blood Sugar Control

The paleo diet, which emphasizes whole foods such as lean meats, fish, fruits, vegetables, nuts, and seeds while excluding processed foods, grains, and refined sugars, can potentially contribute to improved blood sugar control. By focusing on nutrient-dense, low-glycemic index foods, the paleo diet may help stabilize blood sugar levels and reduce insulin resistance. Additionally, the avoidance of refined sugars and processed foods can minimize blood sugar spikes and promote a more stable energy level throughout the day. However, it is essential to consult a healthcare professional before making significant dietary changes to ensure it aligns with individual health needs.

Enhanced Nutrient Intake

The paleo diet, inspired by the dietary patterns of our Paleolithic ancestors, emphasizes consuming whole, unprocessed foods that our bodies are thought to be genetically adapted to. This diet primarily includes lean meats, fish, fruits, vegetables, nuts, and seeds while excluding grains, dairy, processed foods, and refined sugars.

Enhanced nutrient intake can be observed in several aspects of the paleo diet:

Increased Intake of Nutrient-Dense Foods: Paleo encourages the consumption of nutrient-dense, whole foods, including fresh fruits and vegetables. These foods are naturally rich in vitamins, minerals, and antioxidants, contributing to improved overall nutrient intake.

Higher Intake of Essential Fatty Acids: By promoting the consumption of wild-caught fish and grass-fed meats, the paleo diet can lead to

an increased intake of omega-3 fatty acids.
These essential fatty acids play a crucial role in
reducing inflammation, improving cognitive
function, and supporting heart health.

Improved Micronutrient Intake: Nuts and
seeds, which are integral components of the
paleo diet, are excellent sources of
micronutrients such as magnesium, zinc, and
selenium. These elements are vital for
maintaining proper immune function, energy
metabolism, and overall well-being.

More Antioxidants from Fruits and Vegetables:
The emphasis on consuming a variety of fruits
and vegetables in the paleo diet ensures a
higher intake of antioxidants. These
compounds play a significant role in combating
oxidative stress, reducing the risk of chronic
diseases, and promoting overall health and
well-being.

Balanced Macronutrient Intake: While the
paleo diet often emphasizes protein and
healthy fats, it also encourages the
consumption of complex carbohydrates from
fruits and vegetables. This balance of
macronutrients helps regulate blood sugar

levels, providing sustained energy throughout the day.

Elimination of Processed Foods and Refined Sugars: By cutting out processed foods and refined sugars, the paleo diet helps reduce empty calorie intake. This elimination encourages the consumption of nutrient-dense foods, reducing the risk of nutrient deficiencies and promoting better overall health.

Despite these benefits, it's important to note that the paleo diet's restrictive nature may lead to potential nutrient deficiencies if not carefully planned. It is essential to consult with a healthcare professional or a registered dietitian to ensure that the diet is balanced and tailored to individual nutritional needs.

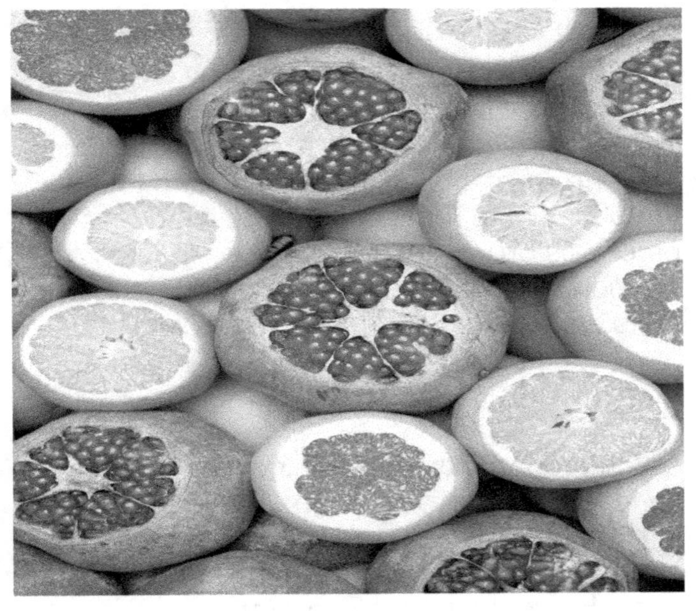

Potential Reduction of Inflammation

The Paleo diet, also known as the Paleolithic diet or caveman diet, is often claimed to have the potential to reduce inflammation due to its emphasis on whole, unprocessed foods. It promotes the consumption of lean meats, fish, fruits, vegetables, nuts, and seeds while avoiding grains, dairy, legumes, and processed foods.

Some proponents of the Paleo diet argue that by eliminating foods that are associated with inflammation, such as processed sugars and grains, it may help reduce inflammation in the body. However, scientific evidence on the effectiveness of the Paleo diet for reducing inflammation is mixed. Some studies suggest that it may have a positive impact, while others do not show significant benefits.

It's essential to keep in mind that the effectiveness of any diet can vary from person to person, and dietary choices should be made based on individual health goals and needs. If you're considering the Paleo diet to reduce inflammation or for other health reasons, it's advisable to consult with a healthcare professional or a registered dietitian to ensure that it aligns with your specific health goals and dietary requirements.

Impact on Metabolic Health

The impact of the paleo diet on metabolic health has been a topic of interest in various studies. Some research suggests that the paleo diet, which typically emphasizes whole, unprocessed foods such as lean meats, fish, fruits, vegetables, nuts, and seeds while excluding grains, legumes, and dairy, may have certain benefits for metabolic health.

Studies have shown that the paleo diet can lead to weight loss, improved insulin sensitivity, and better blood pressure control, all of which are key factors in maintaining good metabolic health. Additionally, the focus on whole foods and the avoidance of processed foods in the paleo diet can contribute to better overall nutrient intake and a reduced risk of developing metabolic syndrome.

However, it is important to note that the long-term effects of the paleo diet on metabolic health are still being researched, and some concerns have been raised about the potential for nutrient deficiencies, particularly in terms of calcium and vitamin D due to the exclusion of dairy products. As with any diet, individual variations and adherence levels can also influence the overall impact on metabolic healthIt is always advisable to speak with a healthcare provider before making big dietary changes.

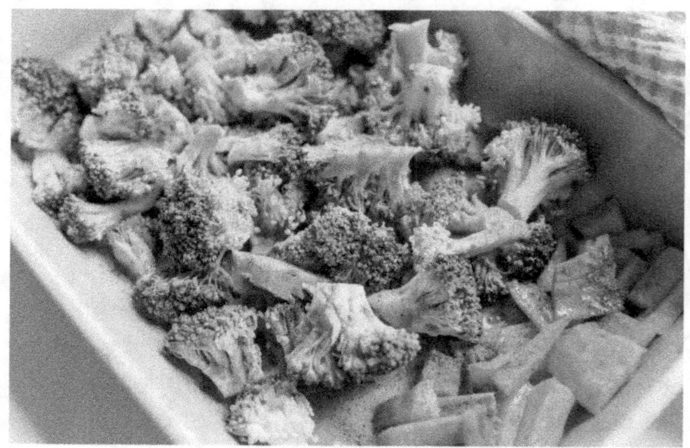

CHAPTER 4

Potential Drawbacks and Criticisms of Paleo diet

The Paleo diet, while popular for its focus on whole foods and avoidance of processed items, has faced several criticisms and potential drawbacks:

Lack of Scientific Consensus: Some critics argue that the diet's historical basis is speculative, and there is limited direct evidence to support claims about our Paleolithic ancestors' diets. Nutritional practices varied widely among different populations during that era.

Nutritional Imbalance: The Paleo diet can sometimes lead to imbalances in macronutrients, particularly with an overemphasis on animal proteins and fats while limiting carbohydrate-rich foods like grains. This can be problematic for individuals with specific dietary needs.

Limited Fiber Intake: The diet's exclusion of grains and legumes can resu t in reduced fiber intake, which may affect digestive health and increase the risk of constipation. Fiber is essential for maintaining a healthy gut.

Inadequate Calcium Intake: The Paleo diet tends to exclude dairy products, a primary source of calcium. This can be concerning for those at risk of osteoporosis or individuals who require higher calcium intake

Sustainability Concerns: The emphasis on animal products in the diet can raise environmental sustainability concerns, as it may result in increased greenhouse gas emissions and land use compared to plant-based diets.

Cost: A Paleo diet can be expensive, as it encourages the consumption of high-quality meats, seafood, and organic produce, which may not be financially feasible for everyone.

Difficulty in Adherence: For some individuals, the strict dietary restrictions can be hard to maintain over the long term, potentially leading to a cycle of dietary fluctuations.

Nutritional Gaps: Without careful planning, adherents may miss out on key micronutrients like vitamin D, iodine, and certain B vitamins, leading to potential deficiencies.

Lack of Personalization: The diet doesn't account for individual variations in metabolism, genetics, or dietary preferences, making it less adaptable for different people's needs.

Risk of Overconsumption: The emphasis on high-fat and calorie-dense foods can result in excessive calorie intake, leading to weight gain if not carefully monitored.

In conclusion, while the Paleo diet has its merits in promoting whole, unprocessed foods, it also has potential drawbacks and has been subject to criticism for its historical accuracy and nutritional completeness. Before adopting any diet, it's advisable to consult with a healthcare professional to determine what's best for individual health and lifestyle.

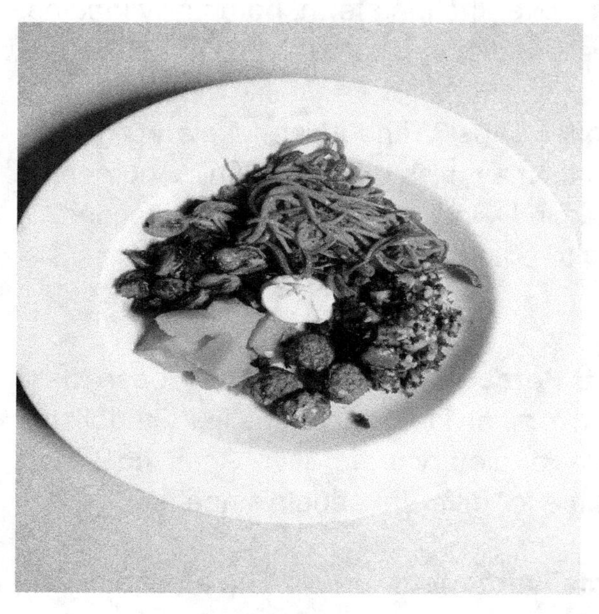

Nutritional Deficiencies and Imbalances of paleo diet

The paleo diet, emphasizes consuming foods that our ancestors might have eaten during the Paleolithic era. While it can have certain health benefits, it's important to be aware of potential nutritional deficiencies and imbalances that can arise from following this diet:

Fiber Deficiency: The paleo diet restricts grains, legumes, and many high-fiber foods. This can lead to a lower intake of dietary fiber, which is essential for digestive health and can increase the risk of constipation and other gastrointestinal issues.

Calcium Deficiency: Dairy products are excluded from the paleo diet, which can result in inadequate calcium intake. A lack of calcium may increase the risk of osteoporosis and bone fractures over time.

Vitamin D Deficiency: Without fortified dairy or other sources of vitamin D, paleo dieters may struggle to maintain sufficient vitamin D levels. This deficiency can affect bone health and overall well-being.

Iodine Deficiency: Since table salt isn't commonly used in paleo cooking, individuals may not get enough iodine, which is crucial for thyroid function. Seafood can be a good source of iodine in the paleo diet, but some people may not consume enough of it.

Vitamin B Complex Deficiency: The elimination of grains can lead to a decreased intake of certain B vitamins, such as folate and thiamine. These vitamins are essential for energy metabolism and overall health.

Iron Imbalance: While red meat is allowed in the paleo diet, excessive consumption of red meat can lead to too much heme iron, which has been associated with health risks. On the other hand, non-heme iron from plant-based sources is limited on the paleo diet, which can lead to insufficient iron intake.

Omega-3 to Omega-6 Imbalance: The paleo diet often encourages the consumption of lean meats and seafood, but not all sources of these foods provide an ideal balance of omega-3 to omega-6 fatty acids. An excess of omega-6 fatty acids in comparison to omega-3 fatty acids can promote inflammation.

Caloric Imbalance: Some individuals may struggle with caloric intake on the paleo diet. The emphasis on high-protein and high-fat foods can sometimes result in consuming too many or too few calories, depending on personal preferences and portion sizes.

It's important for individuals following the paleo diet to be mindful of these potential nutritional deficiencies and imbalances. Consulting with a healthcare professional or registered dietitian can help tailor the diet to meet individual needs and ensure nutritional adequacy. Additionally, dietary supplements may be necessary to address specific deficiencies

Sustainability and Environmental Concerns of the

The paleo diet, while emphasizing whole foods, has been subject to scrutiny regarding sustainability and environmental concerns. This is primarily due to its focus on meat consumption, potentially leading to increased land use, water consumption, and greenhouse gas emissions from livestock farming. Additionally, the exclusion of grains and legumes might contribute to limited crop diversity and increased pressure on specific ecosystems. However, some proponents argue that adopting sustainable and locally sourced animal products can mitigate these concerns. Finding a balance between the principles of the paleo diet and sustainable environmental practices remains a key consideration for its long-term viability.

Exclusion of Dairy and Legumes - Validity and Impact

Exclusion of dairy and legumes from the paleo diet is a fundamental aspect of the diet, and proponents believe it aligns with the presumed eating habits of our Paleolithic ancestors. Here's a look at the validity and impact of this exclusion:

Validity:

Historical Perspective: The paleo diet's exclusion of dairy and legumes is based on the assumption that our Paleolithic ancestors did not consume these foods. While the accuracy of this assumption is debated, it forms the core of the diet's philosophy.

Lactose Intolerance: Some argue that many humans are lactose intolerant, suggesting that dairy consumption may not have been widespread in the past. This lends some validity to the exclusion of dairy from the paleo diet.

Anti-Nutrients: Legumes contain compounds like lectins and phytates, which can hinder nutrient absorption. This is often cited as a reason for their exclusion from the paleo diet.

Impact:

Improved Digestion: Excluding dairy may benefit individuals who are lactose intolerant, as it can alleviate digestive discomfort.

Lowered Inflammation: Some proponents claim that by avoiding dairy and legumes, the paleo diet can reduce inflammation, which may help with certain health conditions.

Potential Nutrient Gaps: Omitting dairy can lead to lower calcium intake, which is essential for bone health. Legumes are a good source of protein and fiber, and excluding them may necessitate finding alternative sources for these nutrients.

Dietary Restrictions: The exclusion of dairy and legumes can make the paleo diet challenging to follow for some, potentially leading to dietary monotony.

In conclusion, the validity of excluding dairy and legumes from the paleo diet is rooted in historical assumptions and the potential benefits of reducing lactose and anti-nutrient consumption. The impact can vary depending on individual dietary needs and preferences, with potential benefits for some, but also the risk of nutrient gaps and dietary restrictions. It's essential for individuals to carefully consider their nutritional needs and consult with a healthcare professional when adopting such dietary restrictions.

Applicability and Challenges.

The paleo diet, which emphasizes consuming foods presumed to have been available to early humans, has gained popularity for its potential health benefits, including weight loss and improved metabolic health. Its applicability lies in encouraging whole, unprocessed foods and limiting refined sugars and grains, potentially aiding in better blood sugar regulation and promoting nutrient-dense eating. However, challenges arise due to the restrictive nature of the diet, making it difficult for some to sustain in the long term. Moreover, ensuring balanced nutrient intake, particularly for essential vitamins and minerals, can be a concern, as certain food groups are eliminated. It is crucial to consult with a healthcare professional before adopting the paleo diet to ensure it aligns with individual health goals and requirements

CHAPTER 5

Practical Tips for Following the Paleo Diet

Some practical tips for following the Paleo diet are:

Focus on whole foods: Emphasize fresh fruits, vegetables, lean meats, and healthy fats while avoiding processed foods.

Meal planning: Plan your meals ahead of time to ensure you have Paleo-friendly options readily available.

Read labels: Be vigilant about reading labels to avoid hidden non-Paleo ingredients in packaged foods.

Cook at home: Prepare your meals at home as much as possible to have better control over the ingredients you use.

Embrace healthy fats: Include sources of healthy fats like avocados, nuts, and olive oil to promote satiety and overall health.

Stay hydrated: Drink plenty of water throughout the day and minimize consumption of sugary beverages.

Incorporate variety: Experiment with different types of meats, seafood, and p ant-based foods to keep your meals interesting and nutritious.

Plan for snacks: Keep Paleo-friendly snacks on hand, such as nuts, fruits, and vegetables, to avoid reaching for non-compliant options.

Practice portion control: Be mindful of portion sizes to maintain a balanced intake of nutrients and calories.

Stay informed: Keep yourself updated on Paleo recipes and meal ideas to prevent monotony and ensure a diverse and enjoyable diet.

Remember that the Paleo diet is ultimately about making healthy choices that work for your lifestyle and goals.

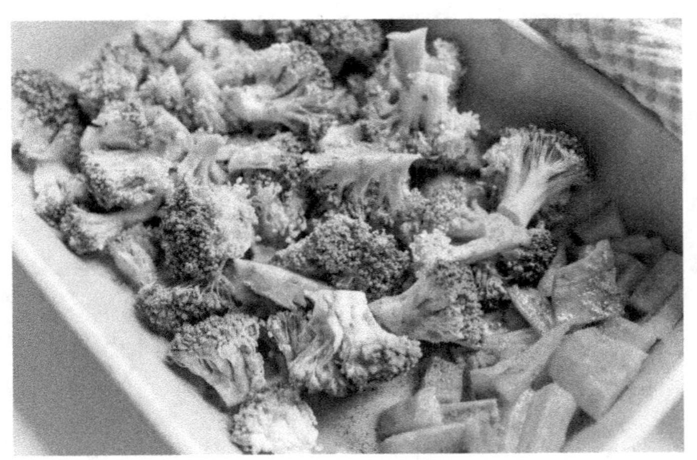

Meal Planning and Preparation

Planning and preparing meals for a Paleo diet involves focusing on whole, unprocessed foods that mimic what our ancestors might have eaten. Here are some preliminary steps:

Meal Planning:

Research Paleo Foods: Understand what foods are allowed on the Paleo diet, such as lean meats, fish, vegetables, fruits, nuts, and seeds. Avoid grains, dairy, processed foods, and sugars.

Make a Menu: Arrange your weekly meal plan. Add a range of veggies, healthy fats, and proteins. Make a shopping list based on your menu.

Portion Control: Pay attention to portion sizes to ensure you're getting the right balance of nutrients.

Meal Prep: Consider prepping some ingredients in advance, like washing and chopping vegetables, to save time during the week.

Meal Preparation:

Proteins: Grill, bake, or pan-fry lean meats like chicken, turkey, and fish. Whenever possible, choose foods that are raised on pasture or fed grass.

Vegetables: Roast, steam, or sauté a variety of colorful vegetables. These should make up a significant portion of your meals.

Healthy Fats: When cooking, use avocado, coconut, or olive oil. Add nuts, seeds, and avocados to your meals.

Snacks: Have Paleo-friendly snacks like carrot sticks, apple slices, or nuts readily available.

Meal Diversity: Don't get stuck in a routine. To make your meals interesting, experiment with different ingredients and recipes.

Avoid Processed Foods: Read labels carefully to ensure you're not consuming any processed or non-Paleo ingredients.

Hydration: Drink plenty of water and herbal teas. Avoid sugary drinks and excessive coffee.

Eating Out: When dining out, look for Paleo-friendly options like grilled proteins and salads. Be clear with restaurant staff about your dietary preferences.

Meal Timing: Some people on the Paleo diet practice intermittent fasting, while others prefer three regular meals a day. Find what works best for you.

Supplements: Consult with a healthcare professional about any necessary supplements to ensure you're meeting your nutrient requirements.

Remember, the key to success on the Paleo diet is planning and preparation. Over time, you'll develop a routine that makes it easier to stick to this way of eating.

Recommended Cooking Techniques

Cooking techniques for a Paleo diet are essential to make the most of this ancestral way of eating, which emphasizes whole foods and eliminates processed ingredients. Here are some recommended cooking techniques for a Paleo diet:

Grilling: Grilling is a popular method for cooking lean meats and vegetables. It imparts a smoky flavor and avoids the need for added fats.

Roasting: Roasting meats and vegetables in the oven can bring out their natural flavors. Use healthy oils like olive or coconut oil for roasting.

Sautéing: Sautéing in a bit of olive or avocado oil is a great way to cook vegetables and lean cuts of meat quickly while retaining their nutrients.

Steaming: Steaming vegetables preserves their nutrients and natural flavors. Use a steamer basket or microwave for convenience.

Baking: Baking is perfect for casseroles, roasted root vegetables, and homemade Paleo-friendly treats using almond or coconut flour.

Stir-frying: Stir-frying with Paleo-approved sauces and lean proteins like chicken or beef can create delicious, quick meals.

Slow Cooking: Slow cookers are excellent for preparing stews, soups, and braised dishes using Paleo ingredients. They're convenient and require minimal effort.

Poaching: Poaching fish or eggs in simmering water or broth is a healthy way to cook and keep foods moist.

Broiling: Broiling is a high-heat method that's great for quickly cooking meats and caramelizing vegetables without added fats.

Raw: Incorporating raw foods like salads, fruits, and nuts into your diet provides essential nutrients and enzymes.

Fermentation: Fermenting foods like sauerkraut and kimchi can be a part of a Paleo diet, as they offer probiotics and digestive benefits.

Sous Vide: This precise, low-temperature cooking method can help you achieve perfectly cooked meats and fish while preserving their natural flavors.

Remember to use Paleo-approved oils like olive, coconut, and avocado oil. Additionally, prioritize organic and grass-fed animal products, as they align better with the Paleo philosophy. Experiment with these cooking techniques to create delicious and nutritious meals that fit within the Paleo framework.

Addressing Common Challenges and Pitfalls of the diet

While the paleo diet has gained popularity for its emphasis on whole, unprocessed foods, it also presents several challenges and potential pitfalls. Some of these include:

Nutritional Imbalance: Eliminating entire food groups can lead to deficiencies in essential nutrients such as calcium, vitamin D, and fiber.

Expense: The cost of adhering to a paleo diet, which often includes organic and grass-fed products, can be prohibitive for many individuals.

Sustainability: The environmental impact of sourcing large quantities of meat and other animal products can raise concerns about the long-term sustainability of the diet.

Social Limitations: Strict adherence to the paleo diet can make it challenging to dine out or socialize, potentially leading to feelings of isolation.

Lack of Evidence-Based Support: While some aspects of the paleo diet are supported by research, the overall diet's long-term health benefits and sustainability still lack conclusive evidence.

To address these challenges, it's essential to consult a healthcare professional or registered dietitian who can help tailor the paleo diet to individual needs and ensure nutritional adequacy. Incorporating a diverse range of plant-based foods, practicing moderation, and staying mindful of environmental and social impacts can help mitigate some of these pitfalls.

CHAPTER 6

Special Considerations and Adaptations

The Paleo diet, based on the presumed dietary habits of Paleolithic humans, emphasizes whole foods, lean proteins, fruits, and vegetables while excluding processed foods, grains, and dairy. Special considerations and adaptations of the Paleo diet may include personalized modifications for specific health concerns, such as:

Nutrient Balance: Ensuring an adequate intake of essential nutrients like calcium, vitamin D, and fiber, which may be lacking due to the exclusion of dairy and grains.

Individual Health Needs: Customizing the diet to accommodate individual health conditions, such as incorporating more sources of healthy fats for those with certain metabolic disorders.

Athletic Performance: Adjusting macronutrient ratios to support the energy demands of athletes while maintaining the core principles of the Paleo diet.

Sustainability: Incorporating sustainable and locally sourced foods to reduce the environmental impact and ensure long-term viability of the dietary choices.

Cultural Considerations: Adapting the diet to include traditional foods and ingredients from different cultures to ensure it is both nutritious and culturally sensitive.

Always consult a healthcare professional or a registered dietitian before making significant changes to your diet, especially when considering specialized adaptations like the Paleo diet.

Paleo Diet for Athletes and Active Individuals

The Paleo diet, also known as the Paleolithic diet or the caveman diet, emphasizes consuming foods that our ancestors would have eaten during the Paleolithic era. For athletes and active individuals, the Paleo diet can provide numerous benefits due to its focus on whole, unprocessed foods.

The diet typically includes lean meats, fish, fruits, vegetables, nuts, and seeds, while excluding grains, legumes, dairy, and processed foods. For athletes, this can lead to improved energy levels, better digestion, and enhanced overall health. Additionally, the emphasis on high-quality protein sources can aid in muscle recovery and development, which is crucial for athletes and active individuals.

However, some athletes may find it challenging to meet their carbohydrate needs through this diet alone, as it restricts certain carbohydrate-rich foods like grains and legumes. It is essential for athletes to ensure they are consuming enough carbohydrates to sustain their energy levels during intense training sessions or competitions.

Furthermore, consulting with a nutritionist or a healthcare professional is recommended to ensure that individual dietary needs, including energy requirements and nutrient intake, are being met adequately. Each athlete's nutritional requirements may differ based on factors such as training intensity, duration, and personal health goals.

Paleo Diet for Weight Loss

The Paleo diet emphasizes consuming whole, unprocessed foods similar to what our ancestors would have eaten during the Paleolithic era. Here's a simple plan to follow for weight loss:

Focus on Protein: Include lean meats like chicken, turkey, and fish. Opt for grass-fed meats if possible.

Abundant Vegetables: Prioritize non-starchy vegetables, such as leafy greens, broccoli, and bell peppers.

Healthy Fats: Incorporate sources like avocados, nuts, seeds, and olive oil in moderation.

Limit Fruits: Choose lower-sugar fruits like berries and avoid excessive consumption.

No Grains or Legumes: Avoid grains, legumes, and processed foods as they are not part of the Paleo diet.

Stay Hydrated: Drink plenty of water throughout the day to maintain hydration and support weight loss.

Moderate Nut Consumption: While nuts are allowed, keep portions in check due to their calorie density.

Mindful Eating: Listen to your body's hunger and fullness cues, and avoid overeating even if the foods are Paleo-friendly.

Remember, individual results may vary, so it's essential to consult a healthcare professional before making any significant dietary changes.

Paleo Diet for Autoimmune Conditions

The Paleo diet, also known as the Paleolithic or caveman diet, is a dietary approach that focuses on eating whole, unprocessed foods that our ancestors might have consumed during the Paleolithic era. It can be beneficial for individuals with autoimmune conditions, although results may vary depending on the specific condition. Consider the following key points:

Inflammation Reduction: The Paleo diet emphasizes the consumption of anti-inflammatory foods such as lean meats, fish, fruits, and vegetables. By avoiding processed foods and grains, which can trigger inflammation in some individuals, it may help reduce overall inflammation, a common factor in autoimmune conditions.

Gut Health: A healthy gut is essential for managing autoimmune conditions, as many autoimmune diseases are linked to gut dysfunction. The Paleo diet promotes the intake of gut-friendly foods like probiotics and fiber-rich vegetables, which can support a balanced gut microbiome.

Elimination of Trigger Foods: The Paleo diet eliminates common food allergens and sensitivities like gluten, dairy, and refined sugars. For individuals with autoimmune conditions, removing these potential triggers can help alleviate symptoms and improve overall health.

Nutrient-Dense Foods: This diet encourages nutrient-dense foods such as organ meats, seafood, and vegetables, providing essential vitamins and minerals that support the immune system and overall health.

Personalization: Autoimmune conditions vary widely, so it's important to tailor the Paleo diet to individual needs. Some individuals may need to make further modifications, such as nightshade avoidance for those with rheumatoid arthritis.

Consult a Healthcare Professional: Before starting any diet, especially for autoimmune conditions, it's crucial to consult with a healthcare professional or registered dietitian who specializes in autoimmune diseases. They can assist you in developing a personalized plan and tracking your progress.

It's worth noting that while the Paleo diet may benefit some individuals with autoimmune conditions, it may not work for everyone. The effectiveness can depend on the specific condition, genetics, and individual responses. It's essential to listen to your body and work with a healthcare professional to find the most suitable dietary approach for managing your autoimmune condition.

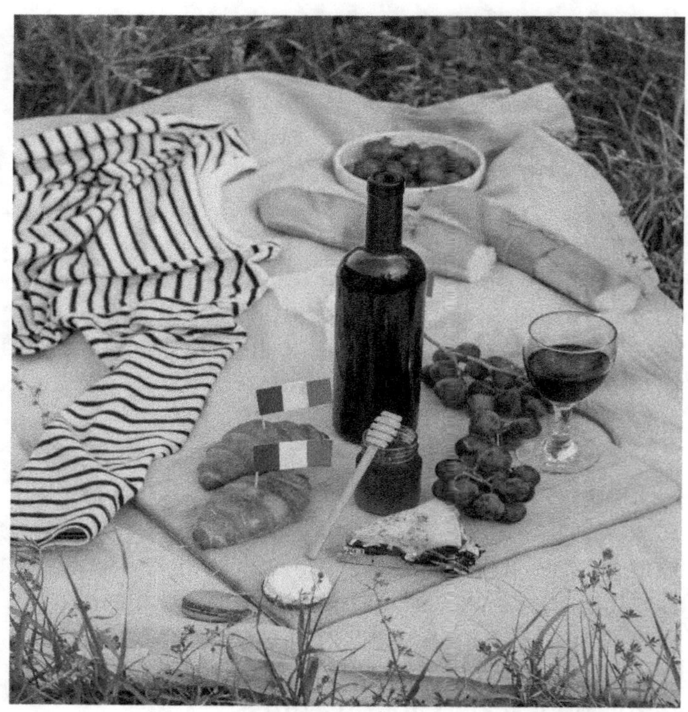

CHAPTER 7

Sample Paleo Diet Meal Plans

Here are some sample meal plans for a Paleo diet. Remember to adjust portion sizes based on your individual needs and consult with a healthcare professional or nutritionist for personalized guidance:

Day 1:

Breakfast: Scrambled eggs with spinach and tomatoes cooked in coconut oil.
Snack: Carrot and cucumber sticks with guacamole.
Lunch: grilled chicken breast with mixed vegetables on the side.
Snack: Mixed nuts and berries.
Dinner: Baked salmon with asparagus and a side salad with olive oil and balsamic vinegar dressing.

Day 2:

Breakfast: Mushroom, onion, and bell pepper omelet.
Snack: Sliced apple with almond butter.
Lunch: Beef stir-fry with broccoli, bell peppers, and coconut aminos.
Snack: Celery sticks with salsa.
Dinner: Baked sweet potato with a serving of roasted turkey breast and a side of steamed green beans.

Day 3:

Breakfast: Smoked salmon with avocado slices and a sprinkle of lemon juice.
Snack: Cherry tomatoes with basil and olive oil.

Lunch: Grilled shrimp with a side of sautéed zucchini and cherry tomatoes.
Snack: Mixed berries and coconut flakes.
Dinner: Grass-fed beef burger with lettuce, tomato, and a side of roasted Brussels sprouts.

These are just a few examples to give you an idea of what a Paleo diet could look like. Remember to prioritize whole, unprocessed foods, lean proteins, healthy fats, and plenty of vegetables while avoiding grains, dairy, and processed sugars. Adjust these plans to fit your dietary preferences and nutritional needs.

Paleo Weekly Meal Plan

Day	Breakfast	Lunch	Snack	Dinner
Monday	Scrambled eggs with vegetables	Grilled chicken salad	Mixed nuts	Baked fish with roasted asparagus
Tuesday	Berry smoothie with coconut milk	Turkey lettuce wraps	Carrot sticks with guacamole	Beef stir-fry with mixed vegetables

Wednesday	Beef stir-fry with mixed vegetables	Tuna salad with mixed greens	Sliced cucumber with salsa	Roast chicken with steamed Brussels sprouts
Thursday	Banana and almond butter	Grilled shrimp with avocado	Celery sticks with almond butter	Pork chops with sautéed kale
Friday	Blueberry and walnut porridge	Vegetable soup with lean beef	Hard-boiled eggs	Baked sweet potato with ground turkey

| Saturday | Scrambled eggs with smoked salmon | Zucchini noodles with pesto | Mixed berries | Grilled lamb chops with roasted cauliflowe |
| Sunday | Paleo pancakes with fresh fruit | Beef and vegetable stew | Mixed nuts | Baked chicken thighs with green beans |

Make sure to drink plenty of water throughout the day and customize portion sizes based on your individual needs and goals.

CHAPTER 8

Resources for Further Information on paleo diet

Here are some resources you can explore:

Books:

"The Paleo Solution" by Robb Wolf.
"The Paleo Diet" by Dr. Loren Cordain.
"Practical Paleo" by Diane Sanfilippo.

Websites and Blogs:

Paleo Leap (paleoleap.com): Offers a wealth of information, recipes, and guides.
Mark's Daily Apple (marksdailyapple.com): Mark Sisson's blog covering the Primal Blueprint, which shares similarities with the paleo diet.
The Paleo Mom (thepaleomom.com): Sarah Ballantyne's website with science-based information and recipes.
Podcasts:

"The Paleo Solution Podcast" by Robb Wolf.
"The Balanced Bites Podcast" by Diane Sanfilippo and Liz Wolfe.

Scientific Papers:

You can explore research articles on topics related to the paleo diet through academic databases like PubMed.

Social Media:

Follow relevant accounts on social media platforms like Instagram and Facebook for recipes, tips, and discussions.
Online Communities:

Join paleo diet communities on platforms like Reddit or specialized forums to engage with others following the diet.

Cookbooks:

There are numerous paleo cookbooks available with a variety of recipes to help you maintain a paleo lifestyle.
Remember to approach information critically and consult with a healthcare professional or nutritionist before making significant dietary changes, as individual nutritional needs can vary.

Cookbooks and Recipes

Certainly! Paleo cooking focuses on natural, whole foods that mimic what our ancestors ate. Here are a few Paleo cookbooks and some common Paleo recipes to get you started:

Cookbooks:

"The Paleo Diet" by Loren Cordain
"Well Fed: Paleo Recipes for People Who Love to Eat" by Melissa Joulwan
"Nom Nom Paleo: Food for Humans" by Michelle Tam and Henry Fong
"Practical Paleo" by Diane Sanfilippo
"Paleo for Beginners" by John Chatham

Common Paleo Recipes:

Grilled Chicken with Vegetables: Marinate chicken breasts with olive oil, lemon juice, and herbs, then grill them alongside a mix of colorful vegetables.

Zucchini Noodles with Pesto: Spiralize zucchini to create "noodles," and toss them with homemade Paleo pesto made from basil, pine nuts, garlic, and olive oil.

Cauliflower Rice Stir-Fry: Pulse cauliflower in a food processor to create rice-sized pieces, then stir-fry with your choice of vegetables, protein, and Paleo-friendly sauce.

Sweet Potato Hash: Dice sweet potatoes and sauté with onions, bell peppers, and ground meat for a hearty breakfast hash.

Baked Salmon with Herbs: Season salmon fillets with fresh herbs like dill and rosemary, drizzle with olive oil, and bake until flaky.

Paleo Smoothie: Blend coconut milk, spinach, berries, and a ripe banana for a nutritious and delicious breakfast or snack.

Remember, Paleo emphasizes whole foods like lean meats, seafood, vegetables, fruits, nuts, and seeds, while avoiding processed foods, grains, dairy, and refined sugars. These cookbooks and recipes can help you create delicious and nutritious Paleo meals.

Paleo-diet Websites and Forums

Some popular Paleo websites and forums include:

The Paleo Diet: A comprehensive website offering information, recipes, and resources for those following the Paleo diet.

Website: The Paleo Diet
Mark's Daily Apple: A blog run by Mark Sisson, covering various topics related to the Paleo lifestyle, including fitness, nutrition, and recipes.

Website: Mark's Daily Apple
Paleohacks: An online community and forum where members discuss various aspects of the Paleo diet, share recipes, and offer support.

Website: Paleohacks
Robb Wolf: Robb Wolf is a renowned figure in the Paleo community, and his website offers valuable information on the Paleo diet, exercise, and lifestyle.

Website: Robb Wolf
These platforms provide valuable resources, recipes, and communities for individuals interested in following the Paleo diet and lifestyle.

Scientific Studies on paleo diet.

The paleo diet has been the subject of numerous scientific studies over the years, examining its potential effects on various aspects of health. Some studies suggest that a paleo diet, which typically includes lean meats, fish, fruits, vegetables, nuts, and seeds while excluding processed foods, grains, dairy, and legumes, may lead to weight loss, improved glucose tolerance, and better appetite management in some individuals.

However, it's important to note that research on the paleo diet has yielded mixed results, and some studies have highlighted potential drawbacks, such as the restrictive nature of the diet and the potential for certain nutrient deficiencies. Additionally, the long-term effects of following a paleo diet are still not fully understood, and further research is needed to fully evaluate its impact on human health.

As with any dietary plan, consulting with a healthcare professional or registered dietitian is advisable before making significant changes to your eating habits. They can provide personalized guidance based on your specific health goals and needs.

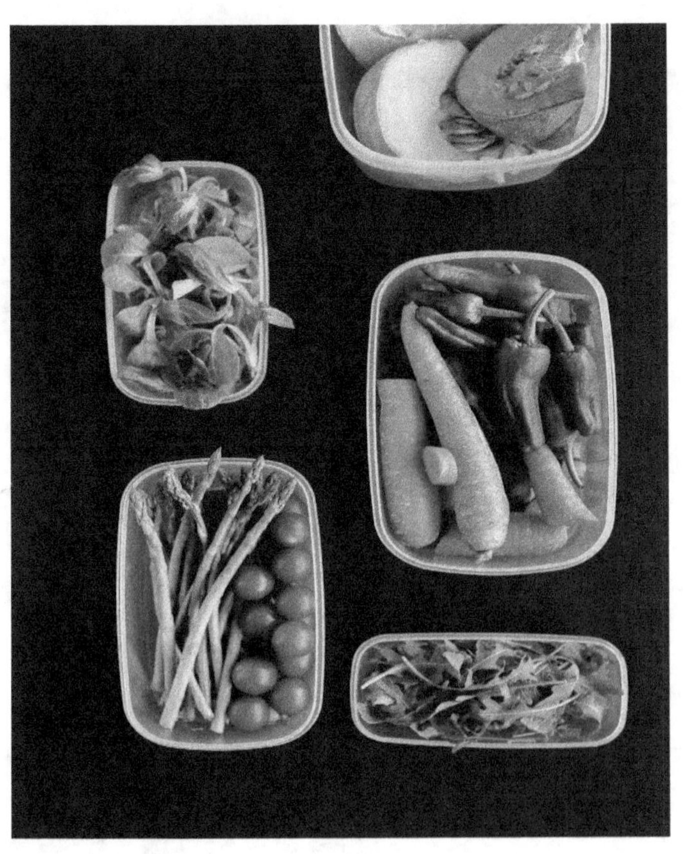

The future of Paleo diet

While it's challenging to predict the exact future of the paleo diet, it's likely that it will continue to be a popular dietary choice for individuals seeking whole, unprocessed foods. As scientific research evolves, there may be modifications or adaptations to the traditional paleo diet, incorporating new insights on human nutrition and health. Additionally, the focus on sustainability and ethical sourcing may become more prominent in the paleo community, reflecting growing global concerns about environmental impact and animal welfare

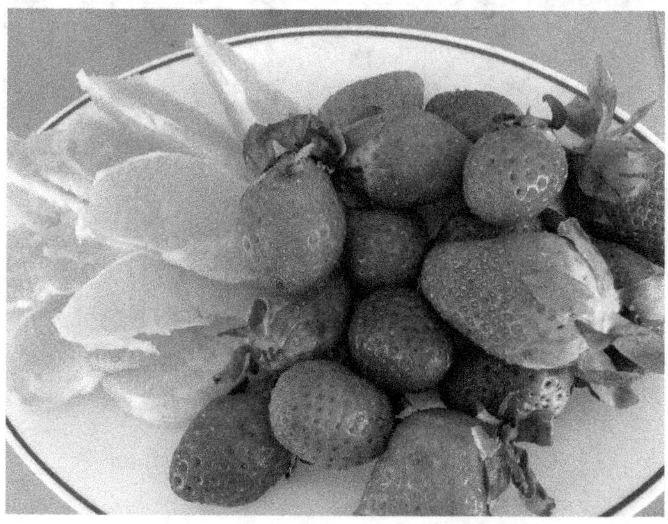

CONCLUSION

In conclusion, the paleo diet food guide emphasizes a return to the dietary patterns of our ancient ancestors, primarily focusing on whole, unprocessed foods such as lean meats, fish, fruits, grains, legumes, dairy, and processed foods while avoiding grains,

legumes, dairy, and processed foods. While it has garnered attention for its potential health benefits, including weight loss and improved metabolic health, the long-term sustainability

and potential nutritional deficiencies associated with the diet warrant careful consideration. Individuals interested in adopting the paleo diet should consult with a healthcare professional or registered dietitian to ensure a balanced and sustainable approach to their dietary choices.